**Published By Robert Corbin**

**@ Cleo Volk**

The Low Fodmap Diet: Delicious Recipes for

Improved Digestive Health and Well-being

**All Right RESERVED**

ISBN 978-1-990666-94-0

I0558142

# TABLE OF CONTENTS

# Kale Salad With Carrots, Almonds & Citrus Vinaigrette

**Ingredients:**

**Dressing**

- 1 tablespoon sherry vinegar, rice vinegar, or red wine vinegar

- Kosher salt

- Freshly ground black pepper

- 3 tablespoons extravirgin olive oil

- 1 tablespoon Dijon mustard, use gluten free if necessary

- 1 tablespoon freshly squeezed lemon juice

**Salad**

- 4 mediumsize carrots, scrubbed or peeled if desired

- 1/2 cup 29 g lightly toasted sliced almonds, natural or blanched

- 1/3 cup 70 g dried cranberries

- 1 navel orange

- 1 pound 455 g washed curly kale, or enough leaves, stemmed and torn into pieces, to equal 1 pound

**Directions:**

1. Prepare the dressing: Combine the olive oil, mustard, lemon juice, and vinegar in a jar and season with salt and pepper to taste. Cover the jar and shake vigorously. Set aside.
2. Prepare the salad: Cut the peel and white pith from the orange.
3. Cut between the membranes to release the segments into a large mixing bowl, reserving all the juice in the bowl as well.

4. Remove any large pieces of kale stem if present.

5. Chop the kale in batches, in a food processor fitted with a metal blade, until finely chopped, adding as it is chopped to the orange segments in the mixing bowl.

6. After all the kale is chopped, remove the metal blade and insert the shredding disk, shred the carrots, then add them to the kale mixture.

7. Toss in the almonds and cranberries. Add the dressing, a little at a time, folding it in.

8. Do not overdress the salad. The kale salad is ready to serve, or refrigerate in an airtight container for up to 4 days.

# Tortilla Baked Eggs

**Ingredients:**

- 1/2 cup baby kale or baby spinach (roughly chopped)

- eggs

- 1 tbsp green onions/scallions (green leaves only, finely chopped)

- cherry tomatoes (cut into quarters)

- 1/8 tsp paprika (small pinch)

- Season with salt & pepper

- 1 tsp olive oil (for brushing the pan)

- corn tortilla (we used Old El Paso Gluten Free Tortillas)

- 1 tbsp colby or cheddar cheese or vegan cheese (optional) (grated)

**Directions:**

1. Preheat the oven to 180ºC (350ºF). Roughly chop the spinach/kale, finely slice the leaves or the spring onion/green onion, cut the cherry tomatoes into quarters, and grate the cheese if using.

2. Grease a small ovenproof frypan or baking dish (you want the dish to be slightly smaller than the tortilla). This Directions: assumes you are making a single serving of the recipe. If you are making more than one serving, then you can either overlap the tortillas in a large dish or use multiple small baking dishes as needed.

3. Gently press the tortilla into the bottom of the dish kind of like you would a sheet of pastry. You want the edges of the tortilla to curl up the sides slightly to form a lip that will hold the eggs.

4. Evenly spread the spinach or kale over the top of the tortilla.
5. Next crack the eggs on top then sprinkle over the spring onion/scallion leaves and chopped tomato. Season with a pinch of paprika and a few grinds of salt and pepper. Then sprinkle with grated cheese if using.
6. Place in the oven and bake for 15 to 20 minutes until the egg whites are set (they shouldn't jiggle when you wobble the pan).
7. Remove the low FODMAP tortilla baked eggs from the oven and slide on to a dish. Cut into quarters and enjoy!

# Chicken Star Noodle Soup

**Ingredients:**

- 2 carrots sliced

- 1 red bell pepper sliced

- Pinch of salt

- Fresh mint leaves for serving

- 1 whole freerange chicken rinsed, giblets, wings, legs and skin discarded

- 1 cup rice star noodles vermicelli or orzo

- 3 big kale leaves chopped into small, bitesized pieces

**Directions:**

**For the Chicken Stock:**

1.  Place the chicken in a large pot over medium heat with enough water to cover the chicken and allow it to slowly come to a boil.

2.  Lower the heat to mediumlow and gently simmer for 1 to 1 1/2 hours, partially covered, until the chicken is done. As it cooks, skim any impurities that rise to the surface; add a little more water if necessary to keep the chicken covered while simmering.

3.  Carefully remove the chicken to a cutting board. When its cool enough to handle, discard the remaining skin and bones and handshred the meat.

4.  Carefully strain the stock to remove any remaining solids.

**For the Chicken Noodle Soup**

5.  In the same pot add the veggies and let them simmered in the broth for about 30 minutes.

6. Add the rice star noodles, shredded chicken, salt and let cook until done (normally 7 minutes).
7. Serve with mint leaves.

# Chicken Pesto Pizza

**Ingredients:**

**Pizza crust**

- 1 1/4 cup + 2 tablespoons warm water 110°F or 43°C

- 2 tablespoons sugar divided

- 1 tablespoon fast action yeast

- 3 cups gluten free flour blend | 420 grams plus more for rolling if needed

- 1 teaspoon xanthan gum ( skip if your GF blend already has xanthan)

- 1 teaspoon sea salt

- 3 teaspoon baking powder

- 3 tablespoons extra virgin olive oil divided

## Toppings

- 1/2 cup low FODMAP pesto

- 2 cups shredded chicken breasts

- 1 1/2 cups | 6 oz shredded mozzarella (use dairy free mozzarella if needed)

## Chive pesto

- 1/2 cup pinenuts

- 1/4 cup nutritional yeast (for dairy free version) or parmesan

- Squeeze of lemon juice

- 1 cup chopped fresh chives

- 1/2 cup fresh basil

- 1/2 cup extra virgin olive oil

- Salt to taste

**Directions:**

**Pizza crust**

1. Preheat the oven to 350°F | 180°C

2. In a small bowl add the warm water and 1 tablespoon of sugar. Stir gently to dissolve the water. Sprinkle the yeast over the top of the water and then stir it in. Set the bowl to the side for 5 minutes to let the yeast activate while you mix together the dry INGREDIENTS:. When the yeast has activated it should foam up a bit.

3. In a large mixing bowl, mix together the flour, psyllium husk or xanthan gum, sea salt, baking powder and remaining 1 tablespoon of sugar. Whisk well to combine.

4. Once the yeast has activated and the dry ingredients are mixed together, slowly pour in the yeast water and 2 tablespoons of olive oil. Mix until a dough starts to form. Lightly flour your hands and a sheet of parchment paper to

roll the dough on and form the dough into a ball. If the dough if far too sticky, add a little more flour a spoonful at a time until it's easier to shape and handle. Depending on the type of gluten free flour blend you may need a little more. Just be careful not to add too much to dry out the crust.

5. Roll the dough into a ball and place in the middle of a sheet of baking paper. Flatten out the dough out with your hands or roll it into shape (about 1/4 inch thick). See notes about rolling. Transfer the dough to a baking sheet and pre bake for 15 minutes. Remove from the oven as your prep the rest of the ingredients.

**Toppings**

6. Spread the pesto over the base of the pizza. Scatter the shredded chicken across the top and then finally top with cheese.

7. Return the pizza to the oven to finish baking for another 1015 minutes. When the cheese starts to turn golden you're done. Let sit for 510 minutes and serve.

**Pesto**

8. Add all of your ingredients to a blender or food processor and process until you get your desired, pesto consistency. You will end up with about a cup of pesto  save the rest for other recipes or top the pizza with more pest at the end.

# Spinach Tofu Curry

**Ingredients:**

- 3 smallmedium sized tomatoes

- 2 inches of ginger root

- 2 cups of baby spinach

- 3 and ½ tbsp of coconut cream

- ½ tsp of turmeric powder

- ½ tsp of pure asafoetida

- 1 tsp of cumin powder

- 2 tsp of garam masala

- 2 tsp of garlicinfused oil

- Salt, pepper, and cayenne pepper

- 5 large leaves of chard

- 2 tsp of sesame oil

- 4 tbsp of green onions/scallions (only use green part)

- 1 small to a mediumsized mixing bowl

- 1 large frying pan

- 1 food processor/blender

- 200 g of firm tofu

- 1 tsp of cumin seeds

- 2 tsp of soy sauce

- 2 tbsp of rice bran, sunflower, OR canola oil (natural oils)

**Directions:**

1. Start by chopping the firm tofu into bitesized pieces and mixing the tofu cubes with soy sauce and turmeric powder in your mixing bowl.

2. Then prepare your ginger and green onions by finely chopping them.

3. Chop the tomatoes as well with less precision since a smallpiece size is not so essential for the tomatoes.

4. Place your frying pan over medium heat and pour your garam masala, asafoetida, and cumin seeds into the pan.

5. Let the spices toast for a few seconds on the heated pan surface and then add in your natural oil so that the spices can fry.

6. Let the spices and oil warm for one more minute before adding the chopped ginger and green onion to the frying pan.

7. Remove the green onions from the pan once they begin to crisp up a little bit and place them to the side.

8. Add the marinated tofu cubes into the same frying pan and cook the pieces until they have a goldenbrown color all around.

9. At this point, remove the tofu from the pan and set the pieces aside as well.

10. Now, add your crispy green onions to your food processor along with the tomatoes, baby spinach leaves, and roughly chopped chard leaves.

11. Blend the INGREDIENTS: until they create a sort of brightgreen homogenous mixture.

12. Add some water to the mixture in the blender, and pour it all out into the hot frying pan.

13. Heat this mixture on medium heat for about 10 minutes.

14. You'll know the mixture is sufficiently cooked once it no longer has a "grassy" aroma or taste to it.

15. When this mixture has cooked for around 10 minutes, add cumin seeds, garlicinfused oil, sesame oil, and coconut cream to the pan.

16. Season this new mixture with cayenne pepper, salt, and black pepper.
17. Add the goldenbrown tofu pieces to the curry in the pan and let everything heat evenly.
18. Serve this curry over a bowl of fresh rice or next to a glutenfree chapati. Enjoy!

# Spinach Eggplant Pasta

## Ingredients:

- 3 tbsp of uncooked tomato puree

- ½ of an eggplant

- Salt and pepper

- 2 tbsp of pine nuts

- 1 tsp of garlicinfused oil

- 2 tbsp of chives

- 1 large saucepan

- 1 large frying pan

- 1 cup of uncooked buckwheat pasta

- 1 cup of baby spinach

- 1 tsp of olive oil

**Directions:**

1. Begin by boiling some water for the pasta in a large saucepan.
2. Place the pasta in the saucepan, along with a dash of salt or according to your preference.
3. Cook the pasta according to the package Directions:, though it generally shouldn't take longer than 10 minutes.
4. Place your frying pan over medium heat and begin to dry toast your pine nuts until they turn a warm golden color.
5. While they are heating, chop up your eggplant into small, bitesized cubes. Once toasted, set the pine nuts aside.
6. In the same heated pan, add your eggplant cubes and cook them dry in the pan over a high flame.
7. As the eggplant is heating, sprinkle some salt over the pieces so that they begin to release some water and brown over.

8. Now, you can add half of the garlicinfused oil and olive oil to the cooked eggplant.

9. Stir fry the eggplant pieces in the oil until they are completely cooked and softened.

10. Bring the heat under the frying pan to low and add your tomato puree to the cooked eggplant cubes in the pan.

11. Stir in your roughly chopped spinach, 1 tbsp of chives, and a tbsp or so of extra water. Allow this mixture to heat evenly, and let the spinach wilt.

12. At this point, transfer your cooked pasta to the sauce in the pan. Serve this pasta in a bowl and top it with the remaining garlicinfused oil, 1 tbsp of chives, and the dry toasted pine nuts. Enjoy!

# Potato Salad

## Ingredients:

- 2 tablespoons chopped fresh parsley

- 85g (1/3 cup) mayonnaise

- 2 teaspoons fresh lemon juice

- Salt & freshly ground black pepper

- 650g (about 5) redskinned potatoes, unpeeled, cut into

- 2.5cm pieces

## Directions:

1. Scrub the potatoes well as you will be eating the skins. Place the potatoes in a pot of cold water and cover. Bring the pot to a rolling boil. Reduce the heat to medium and boil, partially covered for 10 minutes or until just tender. Drain and let cool for 30 minutes.

2.  Place the potatoes in a large bowl with the parsley.
3.  Place the mayonnaise and lemon juice in a bowl and mix with salt and pepper to taste.
4.  Add to the potatoes, being gentle so as not to break the potatoes into smaller pieces.

# Quinoa And Cucumber Salad

## Ingredients:

- 1 teaspoon extravirgin olive oil

- 1/3 cup chopped fresh flatleaf parsley leaves

- 1 small cucumber, peeled, deseeded, diced

- 3/4 cup quinoa, rinsed

- 1 1/2 tablespoons lemon juice

## Directions:

1. Place the quinoa and 1 ½ cups cold water in a small pot over high heat.
2. Cover the pot and bring to a boil, reducing the heat to simmer after the bubbles break the surface.
3. Simmer for 12 minutes until the quinoa is done and the water has been absorbed. Drain and rinse the quinoa.

4. Place in a larger bowl.

5. Mix the lemon juice, oil, parsley, cucumber together in a jar with a lid.

6. Tighten the lid and shake the dressing to combine all the flavors and textures. Pour over the quinoa and toss lightly. Serve.

# Minestrone

**Ingredients:**

- 75 grams shell pasta, glutenfree

- 240 grams carrots, diced

- 12 grams fresh basil, chopped

- 160 grams potato, diced

- 310 milliliters boiling water

- 50 grams celery, sliced

- 160 grams zucchini, diced

- 500 milliliters low FODMAP vegetable stock

- 65 grams middle bacon

- 168 grams canned chickpeas, rinsed and drained

- 80 grams leek

- 2 tablespoons garlicinfused oil

- 400 grams canned plain tomatoes, chopped

- 60 grams spinach, sliced

- 3 tablespoons parmesan cheese

- Olive oil

- Salt and pepper

**Directions:**

1. Remove the white stem of the leeks. Chop the green tips finely and set aside.
2. Slice the bacon into small pieces after removing the rind.
3. Over medium heat, saute carrots, potato, leeks, bacon and celery in a large saucepan using garlicinfused oil for about 20 minutes.
4. Add tomatoes, boiling water, chickpeas, vegetable stock, spinach and zucchini into the

pan. Turn down the heat to mediumlow and let it simmer.

5.  After 10 minutes, put the pasta and basil in the pan. Allow the pasta to cook in the soup.
6.  Sprinkle salt and pepper to taste. Adjust the soup's consistency by adding water, if desired.
7.  Serve with parmesan cheese, baby basil leaves and an extra drizzle of garlicinfused oil.

# Cheesy Chicken Fritters

## Ingredients:

- 2 large eggs

- 2 teaspoons chives, dried

- 60 milliliters mayonnaise

- 2 tablespoons fresh basil, chopped

- 35 grams plain flour, glutenfree

- Olive oil

- 500 grams chicken, ground

- 84 grams mozzarella cheese, grated

- ¼ teaspoon salt

- Black pepper

## Directions:

1. Mix all of the INGREDIENTS: thoroughly in a large bowl. Season with salt and pepper.
2. Place a large frying pan with olive oil over medium heat.
3. Scoop about ¼ cup of the chicken mixture and place it in the pan.
4. Flatten the mixture slightly using a spatula and let it cook for about 4 minutes on each side.
5. Line a plate with paper towel. Once cooked thoroughly, transfer the fritters into the plate to remove excess oil.
6. Repeat the process for the remaining chicken mixture.

# Fried Eggs With Smoked Salmon And Cream Cheese

**Ingredients:**

- Freshly ground dark pepper

- 2 tablespoons unsalted spread

- 8 ounces (225 g) coldsmoked salmon, torn or cut into scaled down pieces, separated

- 4 ounces (115 g) without lactose cream cheddar, partitioned, for example, Green Valley Organics

- 12 huge eggs, at room temperature

- Kosher salt

- Fresh chives

- Fresh dill

**Directions:**

1. Whisk eggs very well in a huge bowl with a sprinkle of water and season well with salt and pepper; put in a safe spot.
2. Melt spread in a huge, nonstick skillet until frothy over lowmedium warmth, whirling it around to cover the container base and up the sides a tad.
3. Include the eggs and cook tenderly for a moment or two, at that point start to get the edges towards the inside as they set.
4. Dab the surface with half of the smoked salmon and half of the cream cheddar and keep on scrambling the eggs until they are light and fleecy yet at the same time a smidgen wet and not dry.
5. Rapidly dab the surface with staying smoked salmon and cream cheddar, include some clipped chives and new dill, to taste, and serve right away

# Quinoa Pancakes

**Ingredients:**

- 1 teaspoon cinnamon

- 1 1/2 cups (260 ml) without lactose entire milk, at room temperature

- 2 huge eggs, at room temperature

- 2 tablespoons canola, sunflower, or vegetable oil

- 1 teaspoon vanilla concentrate

- 2 cups (220 g) quinoa flour, for example, Bob's Red Mill, see Tips

- 2 tablespoons sugar

- 2 teaspoons preparing powder, use sans gluten if following a without gluten diet

- Nonstick splash

**Directions:**

1. Place quinoa flour, sugar, preparing powder and cinnamon in an enormous blending bowl and speed to circulate air through and consolidate.
2. Make a well in the middle and put in a safe spot.
3. Whisk together the milk, eggs, oil and vanilla in a little bowl until very much mixed. Fill well in dry fixings.
4. Whisk everything together just until consolidated  there maybe a couple of bumps and that is alright.
5. Heat electric frying pan, substantial sauté container or nonstick dish, coat with nonstick splash and warmth until a couple of drops of water move.
6. Spoon out ¼ cup measures of hitter at once (we utilize a frozen yogurt scoop) and cook over medium warmth until bubbles start to

show up to a great extent, around 1 to 2 minutes.

7. The bottoms ought to be brilliant dark colored. Flip over and cook for around brief more or until that side is brilliant darker too.

8. Serve hot with genuine maple syrup or potentially organic product whenever wanted.

# Mocha Banana Smoothie

**Ingredients:**

- 1 tablespoon characteristic or Dutchhandled cocoa powder

- 1 tablespoon characteristic nutty spread

- 1 tablespoon chia seeds or flax seeds, discretionary

- Ice 3D squares, discretionary

- 1/2 cup (120 ml) unsweetened almond, hemp or rice milk

- 1/2 cup (120 ml) extremely solid fermented espresso, cold

- 1/3 solidified ready mediumsized banana, cut into pieces

**Directions:**

1. Place every one of the fixings in blender all together recorded and mix until smooth.

2. This beverage is rich! Pour over ice 3D shapes or mix in some ice 3D shapes if you need to weaken it to some degree and include coldness. Serve right away.

# Mixed Salad And Strawberries

## Ingredients:

- 18 g of mozzarella

- 2 tablespoons of vinaigrette sauce

- 1/2 teaspoon of balsamic vinegar

- 100 g of mixed salad

- 80 g of strawberries

- Salt

- pepper

## Directions:

1. Put the mixed salad in a salad bowl after washing and drying it.
2. Add the strawberries to the salad after washing and drying them.

3. Cut the mozzarella into small pieces and add it.
4. Pour the vinaigrette sauce into the salad bowl with the balsamic vinegar and a pinch of salt and pepper.
5. Mix well and serve.

# Roasted Peppers And Tomatoes

**Ingredients:**

- 3 tablespoons of extra virgin olive oil

- 1/2 tablespoon of balsamic vinegar

- 1/2 tablespoon of juice lemon

- 1/2 tablespoon of parsley base

- 1 tablespoon of chives, chopped Salt pepper

- 2 red or yellow peppers

- 3 tomatoes dried tomatoes ( in oil), chopped

- 2 chopped anchovy fillets

- 1.5 teaspoons of capers

- 12 tablespoons of pine nuts (optional)

- 6 black olives

**Directions:**

1. Cut the peppers into quarters and clean them well from seeds and filaments.

2. Place them on the hot barbecue grill with their skin turned towards the grill. after about 5 minutes, turn the peppers and cook them for another 23 minutes

3. . Alternatively, place the whole peppers in a pan and bake for 30 minutes at 220 ° C.

4. After cooking, place the peppers in a bowl, cover them and let them cool for about ten minutes to remove the skin.

5. Then cut them into strips and place them on a serving dish.

6. Add the sliced tomatoes.

7. Drain the dried tomatoes and anchovies, chop them and incorporate together with the capers, pine nuts (optional) and olives.

8. In a cup, mix the oil, balsamic vinegar, lemon juice, parsley base, chives, a pinch of salt and

pepper. Beat with a fork and pour over the

sauce. To serve.

# Grilled Fish With Coconutlime Rice

## Ingredients:

- ¼ small red chile pepper, seeded and finely chopped (optional)

- Freshly ground black pepper

- 4 large boneless, skinless firm white fish fillets (such as snapper or cod; 5½ ounces/160 g each)

- 1½ cups (300 g) jasmine rice

- 3 kaffir lime leaves, very thinly sliced

- ½ cup (125 ml) coconut milk

- 1 tablespoon plus 1 teaspoon fresh lemon juice

- 1 tablespoon plus 1 teaspoon sesame oil

- 1 teaspoon garlicinfused olive oil

- Garlicinfused olive oil

**Directions:**

1. Place all the ingredients for the marinade in a large glass or ceramic bowl and stir to combine well. Add the fish fillets and toss gently to coat. Cover and place in the refrigerator for 2 to 3 hours, turning every hour to ensure even marinating.

2. Bring a large pot of water to a boil over high heat. Reduce the heat to medium, add the rice and one third of the lime leaves, and cook, stirring occasionally, for 10 minutes, or until the rice is tender. Drain and rinse under hot water.

3. Place the rinsed rice in a bowl and stir in the coconut milk and remaining lime leaves. Cover and keep warm.

4. Brush a ridged grill pan or castiron skillet with the garlicinfused oil and heat over mediumhigh heat.

5. Drain the fish fillets and cook for 2 to 3 minutes on each side, until cooked to your preferred doneness.

6. Serve with the coconutlime rice.

# Baked Atlantic Salmon On Soft Blue Cheese Polenta

**Ingredients:**

**Olive oil**

- 2 garlic cloves, peeled and halved

- ⅔ cup (110 g) coarse cornmeal (instant polenta)

- ⅔ cup (90 g) strong blue cheese (or to taste)

- Salt and freshly ground black pepper

- Four 5½ounce (160 g) Atlantic salmon fillets, skin on, pin bones removed

- 3 cups (750 ml) lowfat milk, lactosefree milk, or suitable plantbased milk

- Green salad or vegetables, for serving

**Directions:**

1. Preheat the oven to 350°F (180°C). Brush a baking sheet lightly with olive oil.

2. Place the salmon fillets on the baking sheet, brush with olive oil, and bake for 10 to 12 minutes, until cooked to your preferred doneness.

3. Meanwhile, combine the milk and garlic in a medium saucepan over medium heat and bring to just below a boil.

4. Remove the garlic with a slotted spoon and discard.

5. Add the cornmeal to the milk and stir until the polenta comes to a boil.

6. Reduce the heat to low and cook, stirring constantly, for 3 to 5 minutes more.

7. The polenta should be the texture of smooth mashed potatoes.

8. Stir in the blue cheese and allow to melt. Season to taste with salt and pepper.

9.  Spoon the polenta onto warmed plates, top
    with the salmon fillets, and serve with your
    choice of salad or vegetables.

# Carrot & Fennel Soup

## Ingredients:

- 1 tbsp dairyfree spread (olive oil spread or butter)

- 2 tsp fennel seeds & 1 ½ tbsp fresh cilantro

- 125ml (1/2 cup) low FODMAP milk

- Season with salt & pepper & 8 slices low FODMAP bread

- 240g (2 large) carrot & 340g potato

- 200 g sweet potato or parsnip & 40g (1/2 cup) leek

- 1 tbsp garlic infused oil & 1 tbsp olive oil

- 750ml (3 cups) low FODMAP chicken stock/vegetable stock

**Directions:**

1. Daintily cut the green suggestions of the leek. Strip and reduce the potato, carrot and candy potato (parsnip) into little pieces.

2. Generally, hack the crisp cilantro.

3. Spot the garlicimbued oil and olive oil in an substantial pan.

4. Over low warmth cook dinner the leek hints for 1 to 2mins, mixing sporadically.

5. At that factor include the potato, carrot, and candy potato (parsnip) to the pot, and cook dinner over low heat for 5mins, blending incidentally.

6. Set up the vegetable or fowl stock if necessary (I broke up Massel Chicken Stock Cube 7's in effervescent water).

7. Add the stock to the pan.

8. Turn up the warmth to mediumexcessive and deliver the soup to a shifting bubble.

9. Put the pinnacle of the pot and enable the soup to stew for 10 to 15mins till the veggies are delicate.

10. Then, melt the without dairy spread (olive oil spread or margarine) in a skillet. Include the fennel seeds and prepare dinner for 1 moment, mixing always. Include the crisp cilantro and cook dinner for a further minute, at that factor expel from warmth. At that factor encompass the new cilantro and fennel seed mixture to the soup.

11. When the vegetables are sensitive, expel the soup from the warm temperature and leave to cool for 10 minutes.

12. Move the soup to a nourishment processor or blender, in clusters if necessary, and process the soup until clean.

13. Wash out the soup pot and later on go back the soup.

14. Over low warm temperature combo in the low FODMAP milk, and season with multiple toils of salt and pepper to flavor.

15. Serve the soup heat with a sprinkle of crisp cilantro and a facet of toasted low FODMAP bread.

# Vegan Coconut Green Curry

## Ingredients:

- 240ml coconut milk & 240ml water

- 1 tsp cumin & 2 tsp ground turmeric

- ½ tsp chili flakes & ½ a lime, juiced

- A handful of cashews (optional) & Fresh coriander (optional)

- 2 tsp coconut oil & 1 inch chunk ginger, peeled

- 2 medium potatoes & 1 broccoli

- 1 courgette & 250g spinach

## Directions:

1. At First, Warmth up the coconut oil in a huge pot on medium warmth.

2. Strip and hack the ginger and add to the skillet together with the turmeric and cumin, before blending and cooking for a couple of minutes until the ginger is delicate.

3. In the interim, strip and cut the potato in 1inch 3D shapes before adding to the container and letting sauté for a couple of minutes.

4. You can include a sprinkle of water or more oil if the flavors/potato begin to adhere to the base of the dish.

5. Cut broccoli into florets and courgette into little lumps and add to the skillet together with the coconut milk and identical measure of water.

6. Cook until the potato shapes are delicate (around 1520 minutes relying upon size).

7. Take out from the warmth, include spinach, bean stew drops and a crush of lime and give it a mix.

8.  Include progressively salt and flavors if necessary before fixing with cashews and crisp coriander.

### Pink Grapefruit, Raspberry & Mint Jellies

**Ingredients:**

- 1 pink grapefruit

- 100g small raspberries

- 2 peaches , peeled, stoned and chopped

- 5 gelatine leaves

- 15g fresh mint , roughly chopped

**Directions:**

1.  Soak the gelatine in a bowl of cold water. Put on the kettle and when it boils pour 1 litre of the boiling water over the mint leaves.
2.  eave to infuse for 5 mins then strain into a large jug.

3. Squeeze the excess moisture from the soaked gelatine then stir it into the hot mint mixture until dissolved. Set aside to cool.

4. Cut the peel and pith from the grapefruit with a sharp knife then cut between the segments to release them, reserving any juice.

5. Cut the segments into about 3 pieces each then distribute the grapefruit, raspberries and peaches between 6 glasses.

6. Stir any grapefruit juice into the mint jelly then pour it into the glasses and chill until set.

# Spicy Salmon & Lentils

## Ingredients:

- 3 tbsp olive oil

- juice of 1 lemon

- 2 large handfuls baby spinach

- 2 tsp curry paste

- 410g can green lentils , drained and rinsed

- 2 salmon fillets, about 175g/6oz each

## Directions:

1. Heat a large, lidded shallow pan over a medium heat.
2. Tip in the curry paste and fry briefly, stirring constantly, until sizzling and aromatic.
3. Add the lentils with about quarter of a can of water and season.

4. Heat until simmering then lay salmon on top, skin side up.

5. Cover and leave salmon to cook for 68 minutes until it feels firm when prodded.

6. While salmon is cooking, make the dressing.

7. Mix together the olive oil and lemon juice and season well.

8. When salmon is cooked lift it out of the pan with a fish slice and set aside.

9. Turn the heat up, stir in the spinach and a third of the dressing and cook until the spinach has just wilted.

10. Spoon the lentils and spinach onto two plates then sit the salmon on top.

11. Drizzle over the remaining dressing and serve.

# Warm Chicken Salad

**Ingredients:**

- 1 tbsp soy sauce (or tamari  glutenfree soy sauce)

- 1 tbsp sesame seeds

- 1 bag of salad leaves

- Cucumber slices

- 2 common tomatoes

- 2 chicken breasts (cut into thin strips)

- 2 tbsps. sesame oil

- 2 tbsps. balsamic glaze

- 16 black olives

**Directions:**

1. To make the chicken, heat the sesame oil in a frying pan and add the chicken strips.
2. Fry until almost cooked and then add the balsamic glaze, soy sauce and sesame seeds.
3. Fry until the glaze has become sticky and the chicken is fully cooked through.
4. Add a little water to the frying pan after you've fried the chicken in order to make a little salad dressing.
5. Place your salad INGREDIENTS: on two plates, put the chicken and croutons on top and drizzle with the glaze before serving.

# Chicken Chimichangas

**Ingredients:**

- 100g grated cheddar cheese (or nondairy)

- 4 fresh common tomatoes (diced)

- 12 tbsps. vegetable oil (for frying the chicken chimichangas)

- 8 corn tortillas (or glutenfree tortillas)

- 3 cooked chicken breasts (thinly sliced)

**Directions:**

1. Build your chicken chimichangas by laying out a corn tortilla, adding grated cheese, sliced chicken, some diced fresh tomato and a good grind of fresh black pepper.

2. Fold the sides of the tortilla so that the edges meet in the centre and then fold the top and

bottom towards the centre so that it forms a
tight parcel.

3.  Get your frying pan hot and add a tbsp of
    vegetable oil.

4.  Once it's hot lay the chimichangas folded side
    down in the frying pan and fry them until the
    base is golden brown and crispy.

5.  Turn the chicken chimichangas over and fry
    the other side too.

6.  Once they're crispy and golden serve them
    with Mexican Rice, salsa, sour cream,
    jalapeños, chopped fresh coriander and salad.

# Cheese And Herb Scones

## Ingredients:

- 1/2 cup (115 grams) cold unsalted butter, cut into small pieces

- 1 cup (230 grams) shredded fresh cheese (cheddar, blue cheese, gorgonzola, etc.)

- 3 tablespoons minced fresh herbs (cilantro, parsley, thyme)

- 1 large egg, beaten

- 1 1/2 cups allpurpose flour

- 1/2 teaspoon baking powder

- 1/4 teaspoon baking soda

- pinch of salt

**Directions:**

1. Preheat oven to 400 degrees F. Line a baking sheet with parchment paper.

2. In a medium bowl, whisk together the flour, baking powder and baking soda. Add the salt and stir to combine.

3. In another bowl, using a fork or your hands, mix the butter and shredded cheese until well combined. Stir in the herbs.

4. Add the wet INGREDIENTS: to the dry INGREDIENTS: and mix until just combined. Don't overmix; you want some visible pebbles in the scones.

5. Scrape the batter onto the prepared baking sheet and use a fork or your fingers to form 12 scones they should be about 2 inches wide and 1 inch thick. Bake for 20 minutes or until

# Chocolate Scones

## Ingredients:

- 1 cup granulated sugar

- 2 large eggs, beaten

- 1 1/2 ounces unsweetened chocolate, chopped

- 1 tablespoon milk

- 1 1/2 cups allpurpose flour

- 1/2 teaspoon baking powder

- 1/4 teaspoon baking soda

- 1/4 teaspoon salt

- 3 tablespoons unsalted butter, at room temperature

**Directions:**

1. Preheat oven to 400 degrees. In a medium bowl, whisk together flour, baking powder, baking soda and salt.

2. In a separate bowl, cream butter and sugar until light and fluffy.

3. Add eggs one at a time, beating well after each addition. Stir in chocolate and milk; mix until smooth. Gently fold in flour mixture just until combined.

4. Do not overmix. Scoop scones by rounded tablespoons onto a baking sheet lined with parchment paper.

5. Bake for 12 minutes or until golden brown.

6. Serve warm or cool on the counter for later.

# Escarole Soup

**Ingredients:**

- 12 ounces escarole, chopped

- 6 cups chicken or vegetable broth

- 2 cups diced tomatoes with their juice

- 1 dried bay leaf

- 1 sprig fresh thyme

- 1 tablespoon olive oil

- ½ cup thinly sliced carrots

- ¾ cup diced potatoes

- Kosher salt and freshly ground black pepper

**Directions:**

1. Heat the olive oil in a soup pot over mediumhigh heat.

2. Add the carrots and potatoes, and sauté until the vegetables are just starting to brown, 3 to 4 minutes.

3. Add the escarole. Cook, stirring frequently, until the escarole is wilted and bright green, 4 to 5 minutes.

4. Add the broth, tomatoes, bay leaf, and thyme sprig.

5. Season with salt and pepper, and stir to combine.

6. Reduce the heat to mediumlow, and simmer until the vegetables are tender and the soup is flavorful, 30 to 35 minutes.

7. Remove and discard the bay leaf and thyme.

8. Serve in heated soup bowls.

# Tomato Bisque

## Ingredients:

- ¾ cup carrots

- ½ cup longgrain rice

- 3 cups diced tomatoes

- 6 cups chicken or vegetable broth

- 6 fresh flatleaf parsley sprigs

- 1 sprig fresh thyme

- 1 tablespoon oil

- ½ cup minced green onions, green portion only

- Kosher salt and freshly ground black pepper

- Minced fresh parsley, chives, or thyme, for garnish

**Directions:**

1. Heat the oil in a soup pot over mediumhigh heat.
2. Add the green onions and carrots. Sauté, stirring occasionally, until the green onions are bright green and the carrots are tender, 3 to 4 minutes.
3. Add the rice, tomatoes, broth, parsley sprigs, and thyme sprig.
4. Season with salt and pepper, and stir to combine.
5. Reduce the heat to mediumlow and simmer until the rice is very tender and the soup is flavorful, 25 to 30 minutes.
6. Remove and discard the parsley and thyme sprigs.
7. Purée the soup with an immersion blender directly in the pot or let it cool for 10 minutes and then purée in a blender or food processor.

8. Just before serving, return the soup to a simmer and stir in the chopped herbs. Serve in warmed bowls.

# Quiche In Ham Cups

## Ingredients:

- 4 eggs, beaten

- 2 tbsp rice flour

- 4 tbsp lactosefree milk, can be substituted with other approved milk

- Pinch of salt

- 6 slices ham, cold cut, rounded

- 1 small bell pepper, diced

- ½ cup spring onion, green tips only

- Pinch of pepper

## Directions:

1. Preheat the oven to 350°F and line 6 muffin tins with the ham slices.

2. Mix together the flour and milk, whisking constantly.

3. Add in the eggs, salt, and pepper, mixing until smooth.

4. Add the spring onion and bell pepper. Pour carefully into the ham cups.

5. Bake for 1520 minutes. It's ready when the quiche is puffy and the ham is crispy.

6. Let cool for 10 minutes then use a knife to carefully lift the quiche out of the tins.

# Cheese, Ham, And Spinach Muffins

## Ingredients:

- ½ tsp xanthan gum

- ½ cup thick Greek yogurt

- ⅔ cup lactosefree milk

- 2 large eggs

- 6 oz ham, lean

- ¼ cup chopped chives

- ½ cup cheddar cheese, grated (set 2 tbsp aside)

- ¼ cup baby spinach, chopped roughly

- 1 cup corn flour

- ¼ cup oats

- 2 ¼ tsp baking powder

- ½ tsp paprika, smoked

- A drizzle of olive oil, used to grease the muffin tins

**Directions:**

1. Preheat the oven to 325°F and place a baking tray halffilled with water on the bottom shelf.
2. In a bowl, sift together the flour, baking powder, and xanthan gum, then stir in the oats.
3. In a smaller bowl, whisk the eggs, yogurt, and milk together, then add in the ham, chives, spinach, and cheese.
4. Make a well in the dry mix and pour the wet INGREDIENTS: into it. Gently fold the INGREDIENTS: together. The dough should be slightly wet but not liquid.
5. Grease the muffin tin and fill with the mixture. Wet your fingers and tap the top of the tin gently to settle the mixture.

6. Top with the remainder of the cheese and paprika.
7. Bake for 2025 minutes.

# Low Fodmap Tortilla Salad Bowl

**Ingredients:**

**Tortilla salad**

- 50 g olives  Green or black

- ¼ cup fresh basil and parsley leaves

- 1 tablespoon garlicinfused olive oil

- squeeze lime juice

- pinch salt

- pinch freshly ground black pepper

- 25 g corn tortilla chips

- optional rocket/arugula leaves  To serve

- optional dried chilli flakes  To serve

- 120 g fresh common tomato

- 75 g grilled red bell pepper  Fresh or from a jar

- 46 g canned and drained lentils

- 15 spring onion/scallion greens

**Avocado dressing**

- 30 g ripe avocado

- 1 tablespoon nutritional yeast

- pinch salt

- pinch freshly ground black pepper

- 65 g coconut yoghurt

- 1 teaspoon lime juice

**Directions:**

1. Thoroughly rinse your lentils and allow them to drain over the sink whilst you prep the veggies.

2. In this recipe, I use grilled red bell peppers from a jar to make it super quick.
3. If you prefer you can grill your pepper from fresh.
4. Halve and deseed a medium red bell pepper.
5. Reserve one half for another time. Place half of the pepper, skin side up, under a hot grill/broiler for 510 mins until the skin blackens.
6. Carefully remove from the heat (I use tongs) and place the pepper into a glass jar and close the lid. Leave it to cool for 10 minutes.
7. Once cool enough to handle, carefully peel off the blackened skin, it should come away from the flesh easily.
8. Discard the skin and dice the flesh.
9. Finely dice your tomato, finely slice the spring onion greens and the olives.
10. Tear the herbs into smaller pieces with your fingers.

11. Measure out 46g of drained lentils and pop them into a mixing bowl along with the tomatoes, pepper, spring onion greens, olives and herbs.

12. Add the garlic oil, lime juice, salt and pepper.

13. Mix everything really well and set it aside whilst you make the avocado dressing.

14. Weigh out 30g of avocado flesh, place in a small bowl and mash with a fork until smooth.

15. Add nutritional yeast, salt and pepper, coconut yoghurt and lime juice. Stir everything together really well into a smooth, creamy dressing.

16. Plate up the salad. I like to add a bed of rocket or other leafy greens.

17. Pour the lentil salad and any juice from the bowl on top of the greens.

18. Crush up the corn tortilla chips (I just use my hands) and sprinkle them evenly over the salad.

19. Drizzle over the avocado dressing and top with an optional sprinkle of dried chilli flakes.

# Vegan Cobb Salad With Tempeh Bacon

**Ingredients:**

**Tempeh 'bacon'**

- 1 teaspoon garlic powder

- 1 teaspoon ground cumin

- ½ teaspoon smoked paprika

- 1 tablespoon avocado oil, for cooking

- 1 package tempeh, sliced into 1/2 cm (1/4 inch) slices

- ¼ cup tamari, gluten free if desired

- 2 tablespoons pure maple syrup

- 1 tablespoon apple cider vinegar

**Red wine vinaigrette**

- 1 large clove garlic, micrograted

- 1 teaspoon salt

- freshly cracked pepper

- ¼ cup red wine vinegar

- ¼ cup avocado or extra virgin olive oil

- 2 tablespoons Dijon mustard

- 2 teaspoons dried oregano

**Salad assembly**

- 2 small tomatoes, deseeded and diced

- 1 cup your favourite vegan cheeze

- 1 avocado, sliced

- ¼ cup minced chives

- 2 hearts of romaine, or one head of romaine lettuce, chopped

- 2 cups diced cucumber

- 1 ½ cups thawed frozen corn

**Directions:**

**Tempeh 'bacon'**

1. In a sealable glass container, whisk up tamari, maple syrup, apple cider vinegar, garlic powder, cumin and smoked paprika. Add sliced tempeh, seal and gently invert to coat tempeh with marinade.
2. Marinate on counter for up to 1 hour or in the fridge for up to a day.
3. When ready to cook, heat avocado oil in a nonstick skillet on medium heat. Fry tempeh until golden brown on both sides, about 24 minutes a side. Remove from heat.

**Red wine vinaigrette**

4. In a jam jar, shake up red wine vinegar, oil, Dijon, oregano, garlic, salt and pepper. Set aside.

**Salad assembly**

5. In a medium bowl, toss romaine with half of the dressing. Arrange on platter.
6. Top with cucumber, corn, tomatoes, cheese, and avocado. Sprinke over chives and remaining dressing and serve.

# Low Fodmap Korean Tacos

**Ingredients:**

**Quick pickled veggies**

- 2 tablespoons freshlysqueezed orange juice (about ½ medium orange)

- 1 tablespoon rice vinegar

- 1 teaspoon grated fresh ginger root

- Pinch of red pepper flakes, optional

- 1 ½ cup (100 grams) shredded red cabbage (about ¼ small cabbage)

- ½ cup shredded or matchstick carrots (about 12 medium carrots)

- 1 teaspoon salt

**Korean beef tacos**

- 2 teaspoons Fody Foods ShallotInfused Olive Oil (or garlicinfused olive oil)

- 1 pound lean ground beef (or turkey)

- ½ cup Fody Foods Korean BBQ Sauce (or 1 batch homemade sauce // see notes for recipe)

- 8 corn tortillas

- Optional Garnishes: fresh cilantro, sliced green onion tops (green parts only)

**Directions:**

**Quick pickled veggies**

1. Place the red cabbage, carrots, and salt in a medium bowl and stir to mix. Refrigerate for 2030 minutes.
2. In a medium bowl, whisk together orange juice, rice vinegar, fresh ginger, and optional red pepper flakes.

3. After 2030 minutes, transfer the cabbage and carrots to a colander and rinse under cool running water to remove some of the salt. Transfer the rinsed veggies to the bowl with the orange juice dressing and toss to mix.

**Korean beef tacos**

4. Heat a large skillet over mediumhigh heat. Once hot, add oil and ground beef. Break the beef into small crumbles and cook for about 68 minutes or until the beef is done; no longer pink, and the edges are browned.

5. Stir Korean BBQ sauce into the cooked beef and simmer until the sauce is warm and thickens slightly, about 12 minutes.

**Assemble the Tacos**

6. Warm the corn tortillas using your preferred Directions:. I like to warm mine in an electric griddle or frying pan until the tortillas just start to brown on one side, flip, and repeat.

7. Assemble the tacos by topping the tortillas with Korean beef, pickled veggies, and optional garnishes. Serve warm.

# Low Fodmap Chicken & Lentils

**Ingredients:**

- 1 cup (64 g) chopped scallions, green parts only

- 1 red bell pepper, cored and cut into ½inch (12 mm) thick strips

- 1 ½ teaspoons ground coriander

- 1 ½ teaspoons dried oregano

- 1 ½ teaspoons smoked paprika

- 1, 28 ounce (794 g) can diced tomatoes

- 1 cup (240 ml) low FODMAP chicken stock

- ¼ cup (56 g) dried red lentils, rinsed

- 3 pounds (1.4 kg) chicken thighs (about 6 pieces), bonein, skin on

- Kosher salt

91

- Freshly ground black pepper

- 2 tablespoons GarlicInfused Oil, made with olive oil or purchased equivalent

- ¼ cup (8 g) chopped flatleaf parsley

**Directions:**

1. Season the chicken on all sides with salt and pepper.
2. Add oil to large, cold, straightsided skillet and place chicken thighs in pans, skinside down.
3. Place over lowmedium heat and cook for several minutes, about 8 minutes or so, or until the skin is crisped.
4. The crisped skin is a must. Flip the thighs over and cook for a few more minutes, then remove from pan. The chicken should be a little more than halfway cooked through.
5. Add scallions and red bell pepper strips to pan and sauté over lowmedium heat for a few minutes or until beginning to soften, then stir

in coriander, oregano and smoked paprika
and cook for 30 seconds, combining
everything well.

6. Stir in the canned tomatoes, stock and lentils,
   nestle the chicken back into the pan, skinside
   up, cover and bring to a boil.

7. Adjust heat and maintain a low simmer for
   about 25 to 30 minutes or until the chicken is
   cooked through and the lentils are soft.

8. Taste and adjust seasoning, if desired. Garnish
   with parsley right before serving.

9. Leftovers can be refrigerated in an airtight
   container for up to 3 days.

# Quinoa With Almonds And Feta Salad

**Ingredients:**

- 300g quinoa rinsed

- 50g toasted flaked almonds

- 100g feta cheese, crumbled

- Handful parsley roughly chopped

- Juice ½ lemon

- 1 T olive oil

- 1 tsp ground coriander

- ½ tsp turmeric

**Directions:**

1. Heat the oil in a large frying pan.
2. Add the spices, then fry for a minute or two until fragrant.

3.  Add the quinoa, then fry for a further minute
    or two until you can hear gentle popping
    sounds.
4.  Stir in 600ml boiling water, then gently
    simmer for 1015 minutes until the water has
    evaporated and the quinoa grains are done.
5.  Allow to cool, then add the almonds, cheese,
    parsley and lemon juice. Serve warm or cold.

# Raspberrycoconut Bars

## Ingredients:

- 1/2 cup macadamia, coarsely chopped

- 1/3 cup pepitas

- 2 tablespoons sesame seeds

- 2/3 cup maple syrup

- 1/3 cup macadamia oil

- 2 cups raspberries

- 2 tablespoons lemon juice

- 1/2 cup white chia seeds

- 2 cups rolled oats

- 1 cup shredded coconut

**Directions:**

1. Place raspberries and juice in a small saucepan over mediumhigh heat.

2. Cook, stirring, occasionally, for 3 minutes or until the raspberries have softened.

3. Remove from heat and stir in the chia seeds. Set the saucepan and fruit aside to cool.

4. Preheat oven to 275F. Grease and line sides and bottom of an 8 inch square cake pan.

5. Place the oats, coconut, macadamia nuts, pepitas and sesame seeds in a bowl.

6. Mix the maple syrup and the oil in a saucepan over medium heat for 3 minutes. Pour over the oats mixture and still together.

7. Spoon half into the square pan, pressing with your well greased hands.

8. Pour the raspberry mix over the oats, then top with the remaining oats. Press well with greased hands.

9. Bake for 50 minutes. Cool on a wire rack then place in the refrigerator for one hour.

10. Remove from the fridge and cut into 16 squares with a buttered knife.

# Crispy Falafel

**Ingredients:**

- 5 tablespoons plain flour, glutenfree

- ¾ teaspoon cumin, ground

- 25 grams fresh parsley, chopped

- 2 teaspoons paprika

- 80 grams leek

- 2 tablespoons garlicinfused oil

- 182 grams microwavable brown rice, precooked

- 120 grams carrots, grated and peeled

- 2 tablespoons olive oil

- 168 grams canned chickpeas, rinsed and drained

- Zest and juice of 1 large lime

- Salt and pepper

**Directions:**

1. Set the oven to 190 degrees Celsius.
2. Prepare a roasting tray lined with baking paper.
3. Remove the white stems of the leek and chop the green tips roughly.
4. Except for the plain flour, blend all of the INGREDIENTS: using a food processor.
5. Once the mixture becomes a smooth paste, add the plain flour and mix well.
6. Use 1 tablespoon of olive oil to grease the baking paper.
7. Form small falafel patties using a tablespoon and place them on the roasting tray.
8. Make sure to allocate enough space between each patty.
9. Coat the top of the patties with olive oil.

10. Place the tray in the oven and cook for about 12 minutes on each side.

# Hawaiian Toastie

**Ingredients:**

- 2 tablespoons green onions

- 2 tablespoons butter

- 30 grams shaved ham, sliced

- 40 grams canned pineapple chunks, rinsed and drained

- 2 slices spelt sourdough or wheat bread

- 35 grams cheddar cheese, grated

- Black pepper

**Directions:**

1. Chop the pineapple chunks.
2. Remove the white stem of the green onions and chop the green tips finely.

3. Spread butter on one side of both bread slices. Place cheese, pineapple, ham and green onions on top of the buttered side of the bread.
4. Season with black pepper to taste.
5. Place the other bread slice on top to completely assemble the toastie.
6. Heat the toastie for about 3 minutes or until it becomes golden brown in color.

# Bacon And Egg Salad

## Ingredients:

- 2 medium tomato

- Garlic Infused Mayonnaise

- 4 tbsp mayonnaise

- 1 tsp garlic imbued oil

- Season with dark pepper

- 2 enormous egg

- 100 g bacon strips

- 30 g (1 cup) infant spinach

- 1 little cucumbers

## Directions:

1. Place the eggs in a little pan of cold water.

2. Heat the water to the point of boiling over medium warmth, enable the eggs to bubble for 2 minutes, at that point turn off the warmth and leave on the component for 10 minutes.
3. At that point evacuate the eggs and spot in chilly water.
4. Strip once they have cooled, and cut into quarters.
5. Permit to cool before placing into the bricklayer containers if conceivable.
6. Cut the bacon into pieces. At that point fry in a medium estimated frypan over medium warmth for 4 to 5 minutes until fresh.
7. Permit to cool before placing into the artisan containers if conceivable.
8. Cut the tomato into little pieces. Strip and daintily cut the cucumber, at that point cut into equal parts once more.

9.  Mix the mayonnaise and garlic imbued oil together until smooth. Include a couple of drudgeries of dark pepper.

10. Place the garlic implanted mayonnaise in the containers first, trailed by the tomato, cucumber, child spinach leaves, hard bubbled eggs, and afterward the bacon.

11. Take to work and appreciate! Keep the plates of mixed greens cool until you are prepared to eat them.

# Crisp Green Bean, Chickpea And Jicama Salad

## Ingredients:

- 1 cup (168 g) canned, depleted chickpeas

- 1pound (455 g) jicama, stripped and cut into matchstick pieces

- Low FODMAP Salad Dressing of Choice

- 12 ounces (340 g) slim green beans, stem end cut and disposed of

- Kosher salt

## Directions:

1. Bring a medium measured pot of water to a bubble and salt gently.
2. Include green beans; alter warmth and stew just until green beans fresh delicate.

3. This will simply be a couple of moments. Deplete and run under chilly water to quit cooking.

4. Meanwhile, flush the chickpeas in a strainer with cool water deplete and pat dry.

5. You can cut the jicama with a sharp gourmet specialist's blade or utilize a mandolin, on the off chance that you have one.

6. Prepare the vegetables together and dress gently with plate of mixed greens dressing of decision.

7. Stripped, the plate of mixed greens will toward the end in the ice chest for as long as 3 days.

# Chicken With Olives, Sundried Tomato, And Basil With Mediterranean Vegetables

**Ingredients:**

- Small handful of basil leaves

- 2 tablespoons olive oil

- Salt and freshly ground black pepper

- Four 6ounce (170 g) boneless, skinless chicken breasts

- 2 small zucchini, thinly sliced lengthwise

- 1 small (80 g) eggplant, thinly sliced lengthwise

- 2 heaping tablespoons pitted black or kalamata olives

- ½ cup (75 g) sundried tomatoes, drained (if packed in oil)

- ½ cup (80 g) kalamata olives, pitted

- 2 tablespoons plus 2 teaspoons balsamic vinegar

**Directions:**

1. Preheat the oven to 325°F (170°C). Line a baking sheet with parchment paper.

2. Using a mortar and pestle, crush the black olives, sundried tomatoes, basil, 1 tablespoon of the olive oil, and salt and pepper to taste into an even paste (it can be as smooth or chunky as you like). If you don't have a mortar and pestle, use a blender or mini food processor.

3. Heat the remaining 1 tablespoon of olive oil in a large frying pan over mediumlow heat. Add the chicken breasts and panfry for 5 minutes on each side, until lightly browned and cooked through.

4. Transfer the chicken to the prepared baking sheet and spoon the olive paste over the top. Cover with foil and bake for 10 to 15 minutes.

5. Meanwhile, to make the Mediterranean vegetables, spray a ridged grill pan or castiron skillet with cooking spray and heat over medium heat. Add the zucchini and eggplant (in batches, if necessary) and cook for 3 to 4 minutes on each side, until tender. Add the kalamata olives and warm through.

6. Lightly drizzle both the chicken and the vegetables with balsamic vinegar and serve together.

# Panfried Chicken With Brown Butter Sage Sauce

## Ingredients:

- 1 tablespoon plus 1 teaspoon fresh lemon juice

- Salt and freshly ground black pepper

- Four 6ounce (170 g) boneless, skinless chicken breasts

- 5 tablespoons (75 g) salted butter

- 2 garlic cloves, peeled and halved

- 20 sage leaves

- 2 teaspoons garlicinfused olive oil

- 2 teaspoons olive oil

- Shaved pecorino, for garnish

- Green salad or vegetables, for serving

**Directions:**

1. Combine the garlicinfused oil, olive oil, lemon juice, salt, and pepper in a bowl.

2. Add the chicken breasts and toss to coat.

3. Cover and refrigerate for 3 to 4 hours or overnight.

4. Melt 1 tablespoon of the butter in a large frying pan over mediumlow heat.

5. Add the chicken breasts and cook for 4 to 5 minutes on each side, until just cooked and golden brown.

6. Meanwhile, melt the remaining 4 tablespoons butter in a small frying pan and cook the garlic until golden brown.

7. Remove the garlic from the pan and discard.

8. Add the sage leaves to the butter and cook until the butter is golden brown.

9. Spoon the brown butter sauce over the chicken and garnish with the shaved pecorino.

10. Serve with your choice of salad or vegetables.

# Chicken Star Noodle Soup

**Ingredients:**

- red bell pepper, sliced & Pinch of salt

- Fresh mint leaves for serving

- Whole freerange chicken, rinsed, giblets, wings, legs and skin discarded

- big kale leaves, chopped into small, bitesized pieces

- cup of rice star noodles (vermicelli) & 2 carrots, sliced

**Directions:**

**For the Chicken Stock:**

1. Spot the chicken in a huge pot over medium warmth with enough water to cover the chicken and enable it to gradually reach boiling point.

2. Lower the warmth to mediumlow and delicately stew for 1 to 1½ hours, in part secured, until the chicken is finished.

3. As it cooks, skim any contaminations that ascent to the surface; includes somewhat more water if important to keep the chicken secured while stewing.

4. Cautiously evacuate the chicken to a cutting board.

5. At the point when it's cool enough to deal with, dispose of the rest of the skin and bones and handshred the meat.

6. Cautiously strain the stock to evacuate any outstanding solids.

**For the Chicken Noodle Soup**

7. In a similar pot include the veggies and let them stewed in the soup for around 30 minutes.

8. Include the rice star noodles, destroyed chicken, salt and let cook until done (typically 7 minutes).
9. Present with mint leaves.

# Greek Rice Casserole With Ground Turkey

**Ingredients:**

**For rice:**

- 1 ¾  cup water & 1  cup basmati rice

- ½  tsp salt

**For casserole:**

- tbsp garlicinfused oil or olive oil & 1lb  ground turkey

- tsp dried oregano, divided & ¾  tsp allspice, divided

- ½  tsp salt, divided & ¼  tsp red chile flakes (optional)

- Black pepper to taste & 2 tbsp unsalted butter

- tbsp plus 2 tsp glutenfree flour blend

- 5oz  baby spinach leaves, roughly chopped

- 14.5 oz can diced tomatoes, drained

- cups lactosefree milk & ½ cup pitted kalamata olives, chopped

- Zest of 1 lemon & 4oz feta cheese, chopped

- Chopped Italian parsley for garnish

- Optional for serving: lemon wedges and lowFODMAP hot sauce

**Directions:**

1. Preheat broiler to 375F. Heat the water to the point of boiling in a medium pan.
2. Blend in the rice and 1/2 tsp of the salt.
3. At the point when water comes back to a bubble, lessen warmth to the most minimal setting, spread and stew for 15 minutes or until simply delicate.
4. Expel from warmth, keep secured and rest for 10 minutes.

5. Warmth a huge skillet on medium to mediumhigh warm.

6. Include garlic oil and warmth just until oil is sparkling (don't allow it to smoke). Include turkey and cook, disintegrating with a spatula, until never again pink, 6 to 7 minutes.

7. During the latest possible time or two, mix in 1/2 tsp of the oregano, 1/4 tsp of the allspice, 1/4 tsp of the salt, red bean stew chips if utilizing, and dark pepper to taste. Put in a safe spot.

8. In a huge pot, dissolve the margarine on medium warmth. Include the flour and blend until completely saturated, around 1 moment.

9. Gradually include around 1/2 cup of the milk as you mix. When it begins to stew, include another 1/2 cup while blending and scratching any bits of flour from the edges of the skillet.

10. Change to a whisk and gradually include the remainder of the milk in 2 increases as you

whisk, giving it a chance to go to a stew each time.

11. Proceed to whisk and stew until blend is somewhat thickened 2 to 3 minutes.

12. Go through the speed to break the same number of clusters of flour as you can, yet some little bunches will remain, and that is alright.

13. Lessen warmth to the most reduced setting. Include the spinach leaves, staying 1/2 tsp oregano, 1/2 tsp allspice, 1/4 tsp salt, and dark pepper to taste.

14. Mix until spinach is simply withered, around 2 minutes. Include tomatoes, olives, lemon getupandgo, and ground turkey and blend until simply warmed through 1 to 2 minutes. Mix in the rice.

15. Move to a roughly 2 1/2quart heating dish (11 x 7" or enormous round dish will work). Sprinkle feta on top.

16. Prepare in the focal point of the stove at 375F until fluid is rising around the edges and cheddar is beginning to turn brilliant darker, 20 to 24 minutes.

17. Rest 10 minutes, sprinkle with parsley and present with lemon wedges and additionally hot sauce if utilizing.

# Chicken, Broccoli & Beetroot Salad With Avocado Pesto

## Ingredients:

- 1 tsp nigella seeds

- For the avocado pesto

- Small pack basil

- 1 avocado

- ½ garlic cloves , crushed

- 25g walnut halves , crumbled

- 1 tbsp rapeseed oil

- 250g thinstemmed broccoli

- 2 tsp rapeseed oil

- 3 skinless chicken breasts

- 1 red onion , thinly sliced

- 100g bag watercress

- 2 raw beetroots (about 175g), peeled and julienned or grated

- Juice and zest 1 lemon

**Directions:**

1. Bring a large pan of water to the boil, add the broccoli and cook for 2 mins. Drain, then refresh under cold water. Heat a griddle pan, toss the broccoli in 1⁄2 tsp of the rapeseed oil and griddle for 23 mins, turning, until a little charred. Set aside to cool. Brush the chicken with the remaining oil and season. Griddle for 34 mins each side or until cooked through. Leave to cool, then slice or shred into chunky pieces.

2. Next, make the pesto. Pick the leaves from the basil and set aside a handful to top the salad. Put the rest in the small bowl of a food processor. Scoop the flesh from the avocado

and add to the food processor with the garlic, walnuts, oil, 1 tbsp lemon juice, 23 tbsp cold water and some seasoning. Blitz until smooth, then transfer to a small serving dish. Pour the remaining lemon juice over the sliced onions and leave for a few mins.

3. Pile the watercress onto a large platter. Toss through the broccoli and onion, along with the lemon juice they were soaked in. Top with the beetroot, but don't mix it in, and the chicken. Scatter over the reserved basil leaves, the lemon zest and nigella seeds, then serve with the avocado pesto.

# The Ultimate Makeover: Chicken Pie

**Ingredients:**

**For the filling**

- 4 skinless chicken breasts, 500g/1lb 2oz total weight

- 225g leeks, sliced

- 2 tbsp cornflour, mixed with 2 tbsp water

- 3 tbsp crème fraîche

- 1 heaped tsp Dijon mustard

- 1 heaped tbsp chopped flatleaf or curly parsley

- 450ml chicken stock, from a cube (I use Kallo, organic)

- 100ml white wine

- 2 garlic cloves, finely chopped

- 3 thyme sprigs

- 1 tarragon sprig, plus 1 tbsp chopped tarragon leaves

- 225g carrots, cut into batons

**For the topping**

- 70g filo pastry (I used three 39 x 30cm sheets)

- 1 tbsp rapeseed oil

**Directions:**

1. Pour the stock and wine into a large, wide frying pan. Add the garlic, thyme, tarragon sprig and carrots, bring to the boil then lower the heat and simmer for 3 mins.

2. Lay the chicken in the stock, grind over some pepper, cover and simmer for 5 mins.

3. Scatter the leek slices over the chicken, cover again then gently simmer for 10 more mins, so the leeks can steam while the chicken cooks.

4. Remove from the heat and let the chicken sit in the stock for about 15 mins, so it keeps moist while cooling slightly.

5. Strain the stock into a jug  you should have 500ml (if not, make up with water). Tip the chicken and veg into a 1.5 litre pie dish and discard the herb sprigs. Pour the stock back into the sauté pan, then slowly pour in the cornflour mix.

6. Return the pan to the heat and bring to the boil, stirring constantly, until thickened.

7. Remove from the heat and stir in the crème fraîche, mustard, chopped tarragon and parsley. Season with pepper. Heat oven to 200C/180C fan/gas 6.

8. Tear or cut the chicken into chunky shreds. Pour the sauce over the chicken mixture, then stir everything together.

9. Cut each sheet of filo into 4 squares or rectangles.

10. Layer them on top of the filling, brushing each sheet with some of the oil as you go. Lightly scrunch up the filo so it doesn't lie completely flat and tuck the edges into the sides of the dish, or lay them on the edges if the dish has a rim.
11. Grind over a little pepper, place the dish on a baking sheet, then bake for 2025 mins until the pastry is golden and the sauce is bubbling. Serve immediately.

# Mexican Bean Burritos

**Ingredients:**

- 2 tsps. dried oregano

- 1 tsp ground cumin

- 1 small tin of drained & well rinsed butter beans (140g drained weight)

- 360g of chopped tomatoes (juice drained off)

- 1 pouch of long grain microwaveable rice (250g)

- 100g green bell pepper (diced)

- 100g red bell pepper (diced)

- 1 tbsp smoked paprika

- 1/2 tsp salt

- 8 corn tortillas (or glutenfree)

**Directions:**

1. Place all of your INGREDIENTS: in a large saucepan and heat through.

2. Once hot, taste and season if necessary before serving wrapped in the tortillas alongside grated cheese, jalapeños, salsa, guacamole etc.

# Beef Chilli Nachos

## Ingredients:

- 1 tsp cumin

- 1 tsp dried oregano

- 360g of tinned chopped tomatoes

- Salt and pepper

- 450g beef mince (or vegan mince)

- 200g red bell pepper (diced)

- 1 tbsp smoked paprika

- 2 bags of plain glutenfree corn tortilla chips

## Directions:

1. Cook your beef mince in a pan (I dry fried mine, but you could add a little oil if you wanted) and once it's cooked add the red

peppers, herbs, spices and tin of chopped
tomatoes.

2. Cook for ten minutes and then taste for
seasoning.

3. Add salt and pepper as you see fit, but
remember that your tortillas chips are salted,
so you might not need as much salt as you
think.

4. Put the tortilla chips on each plate and top
with a generous helping of beef chilli.

5. Add any additional toppings and serve.

# Blueberry Pancakes

## Ingredients:

- 1/4 teaspoon baking soda

- 2 tablespoons unsalted butter, melted

- 1 large egg, beaten

- 1 cup blueberries, fresh or frozen

- 1 cup allpurpose flour

- 1/2 teaspoon baking powder

- pinch of salt

- 3 tablespoons sugar

## Directions:

1. Preheat oven to 400 degrees F (200 degrees C).

2. In a medium bowl, whisk together flour, baking powder and salt.

3. In another medium bowl, whisk together sugar and baking soda. Add melted butter and eggs; mix until well combined. Stir in blueberries.

4. Pour batter by 1/4 cupfuls onto a lightly floured griddle or large nonstick skillet; cook for 2 to 3 minutes per side, or until golden brown. Serve hot with maple syrup, if desired.

# Pumpkin

**Ingredients:**

- 1 teaspoon ground cinnamon

- 1/4 teaspoon ground nutmeg

- 1/4 teaspoon ground ginger

- 1 can pumpkin puree

- 1/2 cup brown sugar

- 1/2 cup granulated sugar

- pinch of salt

**Directions:**

1. Preheat oven to 375 degrees F (190 degrees C). Grease a 9x13 inch baking dish.
2. In a large bowl, combine the pumpkin puree, brown sugar, granulated sugar, cinnamon,

nutmeg, ginger, and salt. Pour into the baking dish.

3. Bake for 45 minutes or until a toothpick inserted into the center comes out clean. Let cool before serving.

# Minestrone

**Ingredients:**

- 1 teaspoon dried oregano

- 1 teaspoon dried basil

- 1½ cups tomatoes with their juice

- 6 cups chicken or vegetable broth

- 1 dried bay leaf

- 2 sprigs fresh oregano or basil

- 12 ounces chopped fresh kale

- 9 ounces rice vermicelli

- 1 tablespoon olive oil

- ½ cup minced green onions, green portion only

- 1 celery stalk, thinly sliced

- ¼ cup chopped walnuts

- ½ cup grated Parmesan cheese

- Kosher salt and freshly ground black pepper

**Directions:**

1. Heat the olive oil in a soup pot over mediumhigh heat.
2. Add the green onions, celery, oregano, and basil.
3. Sauté, stirring occasionally, until the vegetables are bright green and tender, 4 to 5 minutes.
4. Add the tomatoes, broth, bay leaf, and sprigs of oregano, and stir to combine.
5. Reduce the heat to mediumlow and simmer until the soup is flavorful, 12 to 14 minutes.
6. Add the kale, vermicelli, and walnuts.
7. Simmer until the kale and vermicelli are fully cooked and tender, 12 to 14 minutes.

8. Remove and discard the bay leaf and oregano sprigs.
9. Just before serving, return the soup to a simmer. Stir in the Parmesan and season with salt and pepper.
10. Serve in warmed bowls.

# Tortilla Soup

**Ingredients:**

- 6 cups chicken or vegetable broth

- 6 fresh cilantro sprigs

- Kosher salt and freshly ground black pepper

- 8 ounces shredded or diced cooked chicken

- ¼ cup chopped fresh cilantro

- 1 tablespoon lime juice

- 1 lime sliced into 6 wedges

- 6 yellow corn tortillas, cut into strips

- 1 tablespoon olive oil

- ½ cup minced green onions, green portion only

- 2 teaspoons chili powder

- 1 teaspoon ground cumin

- 1 cup diced tomatoes with their juice

**Directions:**

1. Preheat the oven to 350°F.
2. Put the tortillas on a baking sheet. Bake until crisp and golden, 15 to 20 minutes. Cool to room temperature. Crumble half of the tortilla strips into pieces. Reserve the remaining tortilla strips for garnish.
3. Heat the olive oil in a soup pot over mediumhigh heat. Add the green onions, crumbled tortillas, chili powder, and cumin. Sauté, stirring occasionally, until the green onions are bright green, 2 to 3 minutes. Add the tomatoes, broth, and cilantro sprigs. Season with salt and pepper.
4. Reduce the heat to mediumlow, and simmer until all of the INGREDIENTS: are tender and the soup is flavorful, 25 to 30 minutes.

141

Remove and discard the cilantro sprigs. Purée the soup with an immersion blender directly in the pot, or let it cool for 10 minutes and then purée in a blender or food processor.

5. Just before serving, return the soup to a simmer and stir in the chicken, chopped cilantro, and lime juice.

6. Serve in warmed bowls with tortilla strips and lime wedges.